......

....

....

DIABETES TYPE:

....

IN EMERGENCY CALL:

....

....

....

YEAR:

....

WEEK OF: ....

MON	BREAKFAST	LUNCH	DINNER	BEDTIME
before				
after				
meal / other				

TUE	BREAKFAST	LUNCH	DINNER	BEDTIME
before				
after				
meal / other				

WED	BREAKFAST	LUNCH	DINNER	BEDTIME
before				
after				
meal / other				

THU	BREAKFAST	LUNCH	DINNER	BEDTIME
before				
after				
meal / other				

FRI

	BREAKFAST	LUNCH	DINNER	BEDTIME
before				
after				
meal / other				

SAT

	BREAKFAST	LUNCH	DINNER	BEDTIME
before				
after				
meal / other				

SUN

	BREAKFAST	LUNCH	DINNER	BEDTIME
before				
after				
meal / other				

NOTES:

MON

	BREAKFAST	LUNCH	DINNER	BEDTIME
before				
after				
meal / other				

TUE

	BREAKFAST	LUNCH	DINNER	BEDTIME
before				
after				
meal / other				

WED

	BREAKFAST	LUNCH	DINNER	BEDTIME
before				
after				
meal / other				

THU

	BREAKFAST	LUNCH	DINNER	BEDTIME
before				
after				
meal / other				

FRI

	BREAKFAST	LUNCH	DINNER	BEDTIME
before				
after				
meal / other				

SAT

	BREAKFAST	LUNCH	DINNER	BEDTIME
before				
after				
meal / other				

SUN

	BREAKFAST	LUNCH	DINNER	BEDTIME
before				
after				
meal / other				

NOTES:

WEEK OF: ....

MON	BREAKFAST	LUNCH	DINNER	BEDTIME
before				
after				
meal / other				

TUE	BREAKFAST	LUNCH	DINNER	BEDTIME
before				
after				
meal / other				

WED	BREAKFAST	LUNCH	DINNER	BEDTIME
before				
after				
meal / other				

THU	BREAKFAST	LUNCH	DINNER	BEDTIME
before				
after				
meal / other				

FRI

	BREAKFAST	LUNCH	DINNER	BEDTIME
before				
after				
meal / other				

SAT

	BREAKFAST	LUNCH	DINNER	BEDTIME
before				
after				
meal / other				

SUN

	BREAKFAST	LUNCH	DINNER	BEDTIME
before				
after				
meal / other				

NOTES:

WEEK OF: ....

MON	BREAKFAST	LUNCH	DINNER	BEDTIME
before				
after				
meal / other				

TUE	BREAKFAST	LUNCH	DINNER	BEDTIME
before				
after				
meal / other				

WED	BREAKFAST	LUNCH	DINNER	BEDTIME
before				
after				
meal / other				

THU	BREAKFAST	LUNCH	DINNER	BEDTIME
before				
after				
meal / other				

FRI

	BREAKFAST	LUNCH	DINNER	BEDTIME
before				
after				
meal / other				

SAT

	BREAKFAST	LUNCH	DINNER	BEDTIME
before				
after				
meal / other				

SUN

	BREAKFAST	LUNCH	DINNER	BEDTIME
before				
after				
meal / other				

NOTES:

WEEK OF: ....

MON	BREAKFAST	LUNCH	DINNER	BEDTIME
before				
after				
meal / other				

TUE	BREAKFAST	LUNCH	DINNER	BEDTIME
before				
after				
meal / other				

WED	BREAKFAST	LUNCH	DINNER	BEDTIME
before				
after				
meal / other				

THU	BREAKFAST	LUNCH	DINNER	BEDTIME
before				
after				
meal / other				

FRI

	BREAKFAST	LUNCH	DINNER	BEDTIME
before				
after				
meal / other				

SAT

	BREAKFAST	LUNCH	DINNER	BEDTIME
before				
after				
meal / other				

SUN

	BREAKFAST	LUNCH	DINNER	BEDTIME
before				
after				
meal / other				

NOTES:

WEEK OF: ....

MON	BREAKFAST	LUNCH	DINNER	BEDTIME
before				
after				
meal / other				

TUE	BREAKFAST	LUNCH	DINNER	BEDTIME
before				
after				
meal / other				

WED	BREAKFAST	LUNCH	DINNER	BEDTIME
before				
after				
meal / other				

THU	BREAKFAST	LUNCH	DINNER	BEDTIME
before				
after				
meal / other				

FRI

	BREAKFAST	LUNCH	DINNER	BEDTIME
before				
after				
meal / other				

SAT

	BREAKFAST	LUNCH	DINNER	BEDTIME
before				
after				
meal / other				

SUN

	BREAKFAST	LUNCH	DINNER	BEDTIME
before				
after				
meal / other				

NOTES:

MON

	BREAKFAST	LUNCH	DINNER	BEDTIME
before				
after				
meal / other				

TUE

	BREAKFAST	LUNCH	DINNER	BEDTIME
before				
after				
meal / other				

WED

	BREAKFAST	LUNCH	DINNER	BEDTIME
before				
after				
meal / other				

THU

	BREAKFAST	LUNCH	DINNER	BEDTIME
before				
after				
meal / other				

FRI

	BREAKFAST	LUNCH	DINNER	BEDTIME
before				
after				
meal / other				

SAT

	BREAKFAST	LUNCH	DINNER	BEDTIME
before				
after				
meal / other				

SUN

	BREAKFAST	LUNCH	DINNER	BEDTIME
before				
after				
meal / other				

NOTES:

WEEK OF: ....

MON	BREAKFAST	LUNCH	DINNER	BEDTIME
before				
after				
meal / other				

TUE	BREAKFAST	LUNCH	DINNER	BEDTIME
before				
after				
meal / other				

WED	BREAKFAST	LUNCH	DINNER	BEDTIME
before				
after				
meal / other				

THU	BREAKFAST	LUNCH	DINNER	BEDTIME
before				
after				
meal / other				

FRI

	BREAKFAST	LUNCH	DINNER	BEDTIME
before				
after				
meal / other				

SAT

	BREAKFAST	LUNCH	DINNER	BEDTIME
before				
after				
meal / other				

SUN

	BREAKFAST	LUNCH	DINNER	BEDTIME
before				
after				
meal / other				

NOTES:

WEEK OF: ....

MON	BREAKFAST	LUNCH	DINNER	BEDTIME
before				
after				
meal / other				

TUE	BREAKFAST	LUNCH	DINNER	BEDTIME
before				
after				
meal / other				

WED	BREAKFAST	LUNCH	DINNER	BEDTIME
before				
after				
meal / other				

THU	BREAKFAST	LUNCH	DINNER	BEDTIME
before				
after				
meal / other				

FRI

	BREAKFAST	LUNCH	DINNER	BEDTIME
before				
after				
meal / other				

SAT

	BREAKFAST	LUNCH	DINNER	BEDTIME
before				
after				
meal / other				

SUN

	BREAKFAST	LUNCH	DINNER	BEDTIME
before				
after				
meal / other				

NOTES:

MON

	BREAKFAST	LUNCH	DINNER	BEDTIME
before				
after				
meal / other				

TUE

	BREAKFAST	LUNCH	DINNER	BEDTIME
before				
after				
meal / other				

WED

	BREAKFAST	LUNCH	DINNER	BEDTIME
before				
after				
meal / other				

THU

	BREAKFAST	LUNCH	DINNER	BEDTIME
before				
after				
meal / other				

FRI

	BREAKFAST	LUNCH	DINNER	BEDTIME
before				
after				
meal / other				

SAT

	BREAKFAST	LUNCH	DINNER	BEDTIME
before				
after				
meal / other				

SUN

	BREAKFAST	LUNCH	DINNER	BEDTIME
before				
after				
meal / other				

NOTES:

MON

	BREAKFAST	LUNCH	DINNER	BEDTIME
before				
after				
meal / other				

TUE

	BREAKFAST	LUNCH	DINNER	BEDTIME
before				
after				
meal / other				

WED

	BREAKFAST	LUNCH	DINNER	BEDTIME
before				
after				
meal / other				

THU

	BREAKFAST	LUNCH	DINNER	BEDTIME
before				
after				
meal / other				

FRI

	BREAKFAST	LUNCH	DINNER	BEDTIME
before				
after				
meal / other				

SAT

	BREAKFAST	LUNCH	DINNER	BEDTIME
before				
after				
meal / other				

SUN

	BREAKFAST	LUNCH	DINNER	BEDTIME
before				
after				
meal / other				

NOTES:

WEEK OF: ....

MON	BREAKFAST	LUNCH	DINNER	BEDTIME
before				
after				
meal / other				

TUE	BREAKFAST	LUNCH	DINNER	BEDTIME
before				
after				
meal / other				

WED	BREAKFAST	LUNCH	DINNER	BEDTIME
before				
after				
meal / other				

THU	BREAKFAST	LUNCH	DINNER	BEDTIME
before				
after				
meal / other				

FRI

	BREAKFAST	LUNCH	DINNER	BEDTIME
before				
after				
meal / other				

SAT

	BREAKFAST	LUNCH	DINNER	BEDTIME
before				
after				
meal / other				

SUN

	BREAKFAST	LUNCH	DINNER	BEDTIME
before				
after				
meal / other				

NOTES: ....

....

....

....

....

....

WEEK OF: ....

MON	BREAKFAST	LUNCH	DINNER	BEDTIME
before				
after				
meal / other				

TUE	BREAKFAST	LUNCH	DINNER	BEDTIME
before				
after				
meal / other				

WED	BREAKFAST	LUNCH	DINNER	BEDTIME
before				
after				
meal / other				

THU	BREAKFAST	LUNCH	DINNER	BEDTIME
before				
after				
meal / other				

FRI	BREAKFAST	LUNCH	DINNER	BEDTIME
before				
after				
meal / other				

SAT	BREAKFAST	LUNCH	DINNER	BEDTIME
before				
after				
meal / other				

SUN	BREAKFAST	LUNCH	DINNER	BEDTIME
before				
after				
meal / other				

NOTES:

WEEK OF: ....

MON	BREAKFAST	LUNCH	DINNER	BEDTIME
before				
after				
meal / other				

TUE	BREAKFAST	LUNCH	DINNER	BEDTIME
before				
after				
meal / other				

WED	BREAKFAST	LUNCH	DINNER	BEDTIME
before				
after				
meal / other				

THU	BREAKFAST	LUNCH	DINNER	BEDTIME
before				
after				
meal / other				

FRI

	BREAKFAST	LUNCH	DINNER	BEDTIME
before				
after				
meal / other				

SAT

	BREAKFAST	LUNCH	DINNER	BEDTIME
before				
after				
meal / other				

SUN

	BREAKFAST	LUNCH	DINNER	BEDTIME
before				
after				
meal / other				

OTES:

WEEK OF: ....

MON	BREAKFAST	LUNCH	DINNER	BEDTIME
before				
after				
meal / other				

TUE	BREAKFAST	LUNCH	DINNER	BEDTIME
before				
after				
meal / other				

WED	BREAKFAST	LUNCH	DINNER	BEDTIME
before				
after				
meal / other				

THU	BREAKFAST	LUNCH	DINNER	BEDTIME
before				
after				
meal / other				

FRI

	BREAKFAST	LUNCH	DINNER	BEDTIME
before				
after				
meal / other				

SAT

	BREAKFAST	LUNCH	DINNER	BEDTIME
before				
after				
meal / other				

SUN

	BREAKFAST	LUNCH	DINNER	BEDTIME
before				
after				
meal / other				

OTES:

WEEK OF: ....

MON	BREAKFAST	LUNCH	DINNER	BEDTIME
before				
after				
meal / other				

TUE	BREAKFAST	LUNCH	DINNER	BEDTIME
before				
after				
meal / other				

WED	BREAKFAST	LUNCH	DINNER	BEDTIME
before				
after				
meal / other				

THU	BREAKFAST	LUNCH	DINNER	BEDTIME
before				
after				
meal / other				

FRI

	BREAKFAST	LUNCH	DINNER	BEDTIME
before				
after				
meal / other				

SAT

	BREAKFAST	LUNCH	DINNER	BEDTIME
before				
after				
meal / other				

SUN

	BREAKFAST	LUNCH	DINNER	BEDTIME
before				
after				
meal / other				

NOTES:

WEEK OF: ....

MON	BREAKFAST	LUNCH	DINNER	BEDTIME
before				
after				
meal / other				

TUE	BREAKFAST	LUNCH	DINNER	BEDTIME
before				
after				
meal / other				

WED	BREAKFAST	LUNCH	DINNER	BEDTIME
before				
after				
meal / other				

THU	BREAKFAST	LUNCH	DINNER	BEDTIME
before				
after				
meal / other				

FRI

	BREAKFAST	LUNCH	DINNER	BEDTIME
before				
after				
meal / other				

SAT

	BREAKFAST	LUNCH	DINNER	BEDTIME
before				
after				
meal / other				

SUN

	BREAKFAST	LUNCH	DINNER	BEDTIME
before				
after				
meal / other				

NOTES:

....

....

....

....

....

MON	BREAKFAST	LUNCH	DINNER	BEDTIME
before				
after				
meal / other				

TUE	BREAKFAST	LUNCH	DINNER	BEDTIME
before				
after				
meal / other				

WED	BREAKFAST	LUNCH	DINNER	BEDTIME
before				
after				
meal / other				

THU	BREAKFAST	LUNCH	DINNER	BEDTIME
before				
after				
meal / other				

FRI

	BREAKFAST	LUNCH	DINNER	BEDTIME
before				
after				
meal / other				

SAT

	BREAKFAST	LUNCH	DINNER	BEDTIME
before				
after				
meal / other				

SUN

	BREAKFAST	LUNCH	DINNER	BEDTIME
before				
after				
meal / other				

NOTES:

WEEK OF: ....

MON	BREAKFAST	LUNCH	DINNER	BEDTIME
before				
after				
meal / other				

TUE	BREAKFAST	LUNCH	DINNER	BEDTIME
before				
after				
meal / other				

WED	BREAKFAST	LUNCH	DINNER	BEDTIME
before				
after				
meal / other				

THU	BREAKFAST	LUNCH	DINNER	BEDTIME
before				
after				
meal / other				

FRI	BREAKFAST	LUNCH	DINNER	BEDTIME
before				
after				
meal / other				

SAT	BREAKFAST	LUNCH	DINNER	BEDTIME
before				
after				
meal / other				

SUN	BREAKFAST	LUNCH	DINNER	BEDTIME
before				
after				
meal / other				

NOTES:

MON	BREAKFAST	LUNCH	DINNER	BEDTIME
before				
after				
meal / other				

TUE	BREAKFAST	LUNCH	DINNER	BEDTIME
before				
after				
meal / other				

WED	BREAKFAST	LUNCH	DINNER	BEDTIME
before				
after				
meal / other				

THU	BREAKFAST	LUNCH	DINNER	BEDTIME
before				
after				
meal / other				

FRI

	BREAKFAST	LUNCH	DINNER	BEDTIME
before				
after				
meal / other				

SAT

	BREAKFAST	LUNCH	DINNER	BEDTIME
before				
after				
meal / other				

SUN

	BREAKFAST	LUNCH	DINNER	BEDTIME
before				
after				
meal / other				

NOTES:

WEEK OF: ....

MON	BREAKFAST	LUNCH	DINNER	BEDTIME
before				
after				
meal / other				

TUE	BREAKFAST	LUNCH	DINNER	BEDTIME
before				
after				
meal / other				

WED	BREAKFAST	LUNCH	DINNER	BEDTIME
before				
after				
meal / other				

THU	BREAKFAST	LUNCH	DINNER	BEDTIME
before				
after				
meal / other				

FRI	BREAKFAST	LUNCH	DINNER	BEDTIME
before				
after				
meal / other				

SAT	BREAKFAST	LUNCH	DINNER	BEDTIME
before				
after				
meal / other				

SUN	BREAKFAST	LUNCH	DINNER	BEDTIME
before				
after				
meal / other				

NOTES:

WEEK OF: ....

MON	BREAKFAST	LUNCH	DINNER	BEDTIME
before				
after				
meal / other				

TUE	BREAKFAST	LUNCH	DINNER	BEDTIME
before				
after				
meal / other				

WED	BREAKFAST	LUNCH	DINNER	BEDTIME
before				
after				
meal / other				

THU	BREAKFAST	LUNCH	DINNER	BEDTIME
before				
after				
meal / other				

FRI	BREAKFAST	LUNCH	DINNER	BEDTIME
before				
after				
meal / other				

SAT	BREAKFAST	LUNCH	DINNER	BEDTIME
before				
after				
meal / other				

SUN	BREAKFAST	LUNCH	DINNER	BEDTIME
before				
after				
meal / other				

NOTES:

WEEK OF: ....

MON	BREAKFAST	LUNCH	DINNER	BEDTIME
before				
after				
meal / other				

TUE	BREAKFAST	LUNCH	DINNER	BEDTIME
before				
after				
meal / other				

WED	BREAKFAST	LUNCH	DINNER	BEDTIME
before				
after				
meal / other				

THU	BREAKFAST	LUNCH	DINNER	BEDTIME
before				
after				
meal / other				

FRI	BREAKFAST	LUNCH	DINNER	BEDTIME
before				
after				
meal / other				

SAT	BREAKFAST	LUNCH	DINNER	BEDTIME
before				
after				
meal / other				

SUN	BREAKFAST	LUNCH	DINNER	BEDTIME
before				
after				
meal / other				

OTES:

WEEK OF: ....

MON	BREAKFAST	LUNCH	DINNER	BEDTIME
before				
after				
meal / other				

TUE	BREAKFAST	LUNCH	DINNER	BEDTIME
before				
after				
meal / other				

WED	BREAKFAST	LUNCH	DINNER	BEDTIME
before				
after				
meal / other				

THU	BREAKFAST	LUNCH	DINNER	BEDTIME
before				
after				
meal / other				

FRI

	BREAKFAST	LUNCH	DINNER	BEDTIME
before				
after				
meal / other				

SAT

	BREAKFAST	LUNCH	DINNER	BEDTIME
before				
after				
meal / other				

SUN

	BREAKFAST	LUNCH	DINNER	BEDTIME
before				
after				
meal / other				

NOTES:

WEEK OF: ....

MON	BREAKFAST	LUNCH	DINNER	BEDTIME
before				
after				
meal / other				

TUE	BREAKFAST	LUNCH	DINNER	BEDTIME
before				
after				
meal / other				

WED	BREAKFAST	LUNCH	DINNER	BEDTIME
before				
after				
meal / other				

THU	BREAKFAST	LUNCH	DINNER	BEDTIME
before				
after				
meal / other				

FRI

	BREAKFAST	LUNCH	DINNER	BEDTIME
before				
after				
meal / other				

SAT

	BREAKFAST	LUNCH	DINNER	BEDTIME
before				
after				
meal / other				

SUN

	BREAKFAST	LUNCH	DINNER	BEDTIME
before				
after				
meal / other				

NOTES:

WEEK OF: ....

MON	BREAKFAST	LUNCH	DINNER	BEDTIME
before				
after				
meal / other				

TUE	BREAKFAST	LUNCH	DINNER	BEDTIME
before				
after				
meal / other				

WED	BREAKFAST	LUNCH	DINNER	BEDTIME
before				
after				
meal / other				

THU	BREAKFAST	LUNCH	DINNER	BEDTIME
before				
after				
meal / other				

FRI

	BREAKFAST	LUNCH	DINNER	BEDTIME
before				
after				
meal / other				

SAT

	BREAKFAST	LUNCH	DINNER	BEDTIME
before				
after				
meal / other				

SUN

	BREAKFAST	LUNCH	DINNER	BEDTIME
before				
after				
meal / other				

NOTES:

MON	BREAKFAST	LUNCH	DINNER	BEDTIME
before				
after				
meal / other				

TUE	BREAKFAST	LUNCH	DINNER	BEDTIME
before				
after				
meal / other				

WED	BREAKFAST	LUNCH	DINNER	BEDTIME
before				
after				
meal / other				

THU	BREAKFAST	LUNCH	DINNER	BEDTIME
before				
after				
meal / other				

FRI	BREAKFAST	LUNCH	DINNER	BEDTIME
before				
after				
meal / other				

SAT	BREAKFAST	LUNCH	DINNER	BEDTIME
before				
after				
meal / other				

SUN	BREAKFAST	LUNCH	DINNER	BEDTIME
before				
after				
meal / other				

NOTES:

WEEK OF: ....

MON	BREAKFAST	LUNCH	DINNER	BEDTIME
before				
after				
meal / other				

TUE	BREAKFAST	LUNCH	DINNER	BEDTIME
before				
after				
meal / other				

WED	BREAKFAST	LUNCH	DINNER	BEDTIME
before				
after				
meal / other				

THU	BREAKFAST	LUNCH	DINNER	BEDTIME
before				
after				
meal / other				

FRI	BREAKFAST	LUNCH	DINNER	BEDTIME
before				
after				
meal / other				

SAT	BREAKFAST	LUNCH	DINNER	BEDTIME
before				
after				
meal / other				

SUN	BREAKFAST	LUNCH	DINNER	BEDTIME
before				
after				
meal / other				

OTES:

WEEK OF: ....

MON	BREAKFAST	LUNCH	DINNER	BEDTIME
before				
after				
meal / other				

TUE	BREAKFAST	LUNCH	DINNER	BEDTIME
before				
after				
meal / other				

WED	BREAKFAST	LUNCH	DINNER	BEDTIME
before				
after				
meal / other				

THU	BREAKFAST	LUNCH	DINNER	BEDTIME
before				
after				
meal / other				

FRI	BREAKFAST	LUNCH	DINNER	BEDTIME
before				
after				
meal / other				

SAT	BREAKFAST	LUNCH	DINNER	BEDTIME
before				
after				
meal / other				

SUN	BREAKFAST	LUNCH	DINNER	BEDTIME
before				
after				
meal / other				

OTES:

MON

	BREAKFAST	LUNCH	DINNER	BEDTIME
before				
after				
meal / other				

TUE

	BREAKFAST	LUNCH	DINNER	BEDTIME
before				
after				
meal / other				

WED

	BREAKFAST	LUNCH	DINNER	BEDTIME
before				
after				
meal / other				

THU

	BREAKFAST	LUNCH	DINNER	BEDTIME
before				
after				
meal / other				

FRI

	BREAKFAST	LUNCH	DINNER	BEDTIME
before				
after				
meal / other				

SAT

	BREAKFAST	LUNCH	DINNER	BEDTIME
before				
after				
meal / other				

SUN

	BREAKFAST	LUNCH	DINNER	BEDTIME
before				
after				
meal / other				

NOTES:

MON

	BREAKFAST	LUNCH	DINNER	BEDTIME
before				
after				
meal / other				

TUE

	BREAKFAST	LUNCH	DINNER	BEDTIME
before				
after				
meal / other				

WED

	BREAKFAST	LUNCH	DINNER	BEDTIME
before				
after				
meal / other				

THU

	BREAKFAST	LUNCH	DINNER	BEDTIME
before				
after				
meal / other				

FRI

	BREAKFAST	LUNCH	DINNER	BEDTIME
before				
after				
meal / other				

SAT

	BREAKFAST	LUNCH	DINNER	BEDTIME
before				
after				
meal / other				

SUN

	BREAKFAST	LUNCH	DINNER	BEDTIME
before				
after				
meal / other				

NOTES:

WEEK OF: ....

MON	BREAKFAST	LUNCH	DINNER	BEDTIME
before				
after				
meal / other				

TUE	BREAKFAST	LUNCH	DINNER	BEDTIME
before				
after				
meal / other				

WED	BREAKFAST	LUNCH	DINNER	BEDTIME
before				
after				
meal / other				

THU	BREAKFAST	LUNCH	DINNER	BEDTIME
before				
after				
meal / other				

FRI

	BREAKFAST	LUNCH	DINNER	BEDTIME
before				
after				
meal / other				

SAT

	BREAKFAST	LUNCH	DINNER	BEDTIME
before				
after				
meal / other				

SUN

	BREAKFAST	LUNCH	DINNER	BEDTIME
before				
after				
meal / other				

NOTES:

WEEK OF: ....

MON	BREAKFAST	LUNCH	DINNER	BEDTIME
before				
after				
meal / other				

TUE	BREAKFAST	LUNCH	DINNER	BEDTIME
before				
after				
meal / other				

WED	BREAKFAST	LUNCH	DINNER	BEDTIME
before				
after				
meal / other				

THU	BREAKFAST	LUNCH	DINNER	BEDTIME
before				
after				
meal / other				

FRI

	BREAKFAST	LUNCH	DINNER	BEDTIME
before				
after				
meal / other				

SAT

	BREAKFAST	LUNCH	DINNER	BEDTIME
before				
after				
meal / other				

SUN

	BREAKFAST	LUNCH	DINNER	BEDTIME
before				
after				
meal / other				

OTES:

WEEK OF: ....

MON	BREAKFAST	LUNCH	DINNER	BEDTIME
before				
after				
meal / other				

TUE	BREAKFAST	LUNCH	DINNER	BEDTIME
before				
after				
meal / other				

WED	BREAKFAST	LUNCH	DINNER	BEDTIME
before				
after				
meal / other				

THU	BREAKFAST	LUNCH	DINNER	BEDTIME
before				
after				
meal / other				

FRI

	BREAKFAST	LUNCH	DINNER	BEDTIME
before				
after				
meal / other				

SAT

	BREAKFAST	LUNCH	DINNER	BEDTIME
before				
after				
meal / other				

SUN

	BREAKFAST	LUNCH	DINNER	BEDTIME
before				
after				
meal / other				

NOTES:

WEEK OF: ....

MON	BREAKFAST	LUNCH	DINNER	BEDTIME
before				
after				
meal / other				

TUE	BREAKFAST	LUNCH	DINNER	BEDTIME
before				
after				
meal / other				

WED	BREAKFAST	LUNCH	DINNER	BEDTIME
before				
after				
meal / other				

THU	BREAKFAST	LUNCH	DINNER	BEDTIME
before				
after				
meal / other				

FRI	BREAKFAST	LUNCH	DINNER	BEDTIME
before				
after				
meal / other				

SAT	BREAKFAST	LUNCH	DINNER	BEDTIME
before				
after				
meal / other				

SUN	BREAKFAST	LUNCH	DINNER	BEDTIME
before				
after				
meal / other				

NOTES:

....

....

....

....

....

WEEK OF: ....

MON	BREAKFAST	LUNCH	DINNER	BEDTIME
before				
after				
meal / other				

TUE	BREAKFAST	LUNCH	DINNER	BEDTIME
before				
after				
meal / other				

WED	BREAKFAST	LUNCH	DINNER	BEDTIME
before				
after				
meal / other				

THU	BREAKFAST	LUNCH	DINNER	BEDTIME
before				
after				
meal / other				

FRI

	BREAKFAST	LUNCH	DINNER	BEDTIME
before				
after				
meal / other				

SAT

	BREAKFAST	LUNCH	DINNER	BEDTIME
before				
after				
meal / other				

SUN

	BREAKFAST	LUNCH	DINNER	BEDTIME
before				
after				
meal / other				

OTES:

....

....

....

....

....

WEEK OF: ....

MON	BREAKFAST	LUNCH	DINNER	BEDTIME
before				
after				
meal / other				

TUE	BREAKFAST	LUNCH	DINNER	BEDTIME
before				
after				
meal / other				

WED	BREAKFAST	LUNCH	DINNER	BEDTIME
before				
after				
meal / other				

THU	BREAKFAST	LUNCH	DINNER	BEDTIME
before				
after				
meal / other				

FRI	BREAKFAST	LUNCH	DINNER	BEDTIME
before				
after				
meal / other				

SAT	BREAKFAST	LUNCH	DINNER	BEDTIME
before				
after				
meal / other				

SUN	BREAKFAST	LUNCH	DINNER	BEDTIME
before				
after				
meal / other				

NOTES:

WEEK OF: ....

MON	BREAKFAST	LUNCH	DINNER	BEDTIME
before				
after				
meal / other				

TUE	BREAKFAST	LUNCH	DINNER	BEDTIME
before				
after				
meal / other				

WED	BREAKFAST	LUNCH	DINNER	BEDTIME
before				
after				
meal / other				

THU	BREAKFAST	LUNCH	DINNER	BEDTIME
before				
after				
meal / other				

FRI

	BREAKFAST	LUNCH	DINNER	BEDTIME
before				
after				
meal / other				

SAT

	BREAKFAST	LUNCH	DINNER	BEDTIME
before				
after				
meal / other				

SUN

	BREAKFAST	LUNCH	DINNER	BEDTIME
before				
after				
meal / other				

NOTES:

WEEK OF: ....

MON	BREAKFAST	LUNCH	DINNER	BEDTIME
before				
after				
meal / other				

TUE	BREAKFAST	LUNCH	DINNER	BEDTIME
before				
after				
meal / other				

WED	BREAKFAST	LUNCH	DINNER	BEDTIME
before				
after				
meal / other				

THU	BREAKFAST	LUNCH	DINNER	BEDTIME
before				
after				
meal / other				

FRI	BREAKFAST	LUNCH	DINNER	BEDTIME
before				
after				
meal / other				

SAT	BREAKFAST	LUNCH	DINNER	BEDTIME
before				
after				
meal / other				

SUN	BREAKFAST	LUNCH	DINNER	BEDTIME
before				
after				
meal / other				

NOTES:

MON

	BREAKFAST	LUNCH	DINNER	BEDTIME
before				
after				
meal / other				

TUE

	BREAKFAST	LUNCH	DINNER	BEDTIME
before				
after				
meal / other				

WED

	BREAKFAST	LUNCH	DINNER	BEDTIME
before				
after				
meal / other				

THU

	BREAKFAST	LUNCH	DINNER	BEDTIME
before				
after				
meal / other				

FRI	BREAKFAST	LUNCH	DINNER	BEDTIME
before				
after				
meal / other				

SAT	BREAKFAST	LUNCH	DINNER	BEDTIME
before				
after				
meal / other				

SUN	BREAKFAST	LUNCH	DINNER	BEDTIME
before				
after				
meal / other				

NOTES:

MON	BREAKFAST	LUNCH	DINNER	BEDTIME
before				
after				
meal / other				

TUE	BREAKFAST	LUNCH	DINNER	BEDTIME
before				
after				
meal / other				

WED	BREAKFAST	LUNCH	DINNER	BEDTIME
before				
after				
meal / other				

THU	BREAKFAST	LUNCH	DINNER	BEDTIME
before				
after				
meal / other				

FRI

	BREAKFAST	LUNCH	DINNER	BEDTIME
before				
after				
meal / other				

SAT

	BREAKFAST	LUNCH	DINNER	BEDTIME
before				
after				
meal / other				

SUN

	BREAKFAST	LUNCH	DINNER	BEDTIME
before				
after				
meal / other				

OTES:

WEEK OF: ....

MON	BREAKFAST	LUNCH	DINNER	BEDTIME
before				
after				
meal / other				

TUE	BREAKFAST	LUNCH	DINNER	BEDTIME
before				
after				
meal / other				

WED	BREAKFAST	LUNCH	DINNER	BEDTIME
before				
after				
meal / other				

THU	BREAKFAST	LUNCH	DINNER	BEDTIME
before				
after				
meal / other				

FRI

	BREAKFAST	LUNCH	DINNER	BEDTIME
before				
after				
meal / other				

SAT

	BREAKFAST	LUNCH	DINNER	BEDTIME
before				
after				
meal / other				

SUN

	BREAKFAST	LUNCH	DINNER	BEDTIME
before				
after				
meal / other				

OTES:

WEEK OF: ....

MON	BREAKFAST	LUNCH	DINNER	BEDTIME
before				
after				
meal / other				

TUE	BREAKFAST	LUNCH	DINNER	BEDTIME
before				
after				
meal / other				

WED	BREAKFAST	LUNCH	DINNER	BEDTIME
before				
after				
meal / other				

THU	BREAKFAST	LUNCH	DINNER	BEDTIME
before				
after				
meal / other				

FRI

	BREAKFAST	LUNCH	DINNER	BEDTIME
before				
after				
meal / other				

SAT

	BREAKFAST	LUNCH	DINNER	BEDTIME
before				
after				
meal / other				

SUN

	BREAKFAST	LUNCH	DINNER	BEDTIME
before				
after				
meal / other				

NOTES:

WEEK OF: ....

MON	BREAKFAST	LUNCH	DINNER	BEDTIME
before				
after				
meal / other				

TUE	BREAKFAST	LUNCH	DINNER	BEDTIME
before				
after				
meal / other				

WED	BREAKFAST	LUNCH	DINNER	BEDTIME
before				
after				
meal / other				

THU	BREAKFAST	LUNCH	DINNER	BEDTIME
before				
after				
meal / other				

FRI	BREAKFAST	LUNCH	DINNER	BEDTIME
before				
after				
meal / other				

SAT	BREAKFAST	LUNCH	DINNER	BEDTIME
before				
after				
meal / other				

SUN	BREAKFAST	LUNCH	DINNER	BEDTIME
before				
after				
meal / other				

NOTES:

MON	BREAKFAST	LUNCH	DINNER	BEDTIME
before				
after				
meal / other				

TUE	BREAKFAST	LUNCH	DINNER	BEDTIME
before				
after				
meal / other				

WED	BREAKFAST	LUNCH	DINNER	BEDTIME
before				
after				
meal / other				

THU	BREAKFAST	LUNCH	DINNER	BEDTIME
before				
after				
meal / other				

FRI

	BREAKFAST	LUNCH	DINNER	BEDTIME
before				
after				
meal / other				

SAT

	BREAKFAST	LUNCH	DINNER	BEDTIME
before				
after				
meal / other				

SUN

	BREAKFAST	LUNCH	DINNER	BEDTIME
before				
after				
meal / other				

NOTES:

WEEK OF: ....

MON	BREAKFAST	LUNCH	DINNER	BEDTIME
before				
after				
meal / other				

TUE	BREAKFAST	LUNCH	DINNER	BEDTIME
before				
after				
meal / other				

WED	BREAKFAST	LUNCH	DINNER	BEDTIME
before				
after				
meal / other				

THU	BREAKFAST	LUNCH	DINNER	BEDTIME
before				
after				
meal / other				

FRI	BREAKFAST	LUNCH	DINNER	BEDTIME
before				
after				
meal / other				

SAT	BREAKFAST	LUNCH	DINNER	BEDTIME
before				
after				
meal / other				

SUN	BREAKFAST	LUNCH	DINNER	BEDTIME
before				
after				
meal / other				

NOTES:

WEEK OF: ....

MON	BREAKFAST	LUNCH	DINNER	BEDTIME
before				
after				
meal / other				

TUE	BREAKFAST	LUNCH	DINNER	BEDTIME
before				
after				
meal / other				

WED	BREAKFAST	LUNCH	DINNER	BEDTIME
before				
after				
meal / other				

THU	BREAKFAST	LUNCH	DINNER	BEDTIME
before				
after				
meal / other				

FRI

	BREAKFAST	LUNCH	DINNER	BEDTIME
before				
after				
meal / other				

SAT

	BREAKFAST	LUNCH	DINNER	BEDTIME
before				
after				
meal / other				

SUN

	BREAKFAST	LUNCH	DINNER	BEDTIME
before				
after				
meal / other				

NOTES:

WEEK OF: ....

MON	BREAKFAST	LUNCH	DINNER	BEDTIME
before				
after				
meal / other				

TUE	BREAKFAST	LUNCH	DINNER	BEDTIME
before				
after				
meal / other				

WED	BREAKFAST	LUNCH	DINNER	BEDTIME
before				
after				
meal / other				

THU	BREAKFAST	LUNCH	DINNER	BEDTIME
before				
after				
meal / other				

FRI	BREAKFAST	LUNCH	DINNER	BEDTIME
before				
after				
meal / other				

SAT	BREAKFAST	LUNCH	DINNER	BEDTIME
before				
after				
meal / other				

SUN	BREAKFAST	LUNCH	DINNER	BEDTIME
before				
after				
meal / other				

NOTES:

WEEK OF: ....

MON	BREAKFAST	LUNCH	DINNER	BEDTIME
before				
after				
meal / other				

TUE	BREAKFAST	LUNCH	DINNER	BEDTIME
before				
after				
meal / other				

WED	BREAKFAST	LUNCH	DINNER	BEDTIME
before				
after				
meal / other				

THU	BREAKFAST	LUNCH	DINNER	BEDTIME
before				
after				
meal / other				

FRI	BREAKFAST	LUNCH	DINNER	BEDTIME
before				
after				
meal / other				

SAT	BREAKFAST	LUNCH	DINNER	BEDTIME
before				
after				
meal / other				

SUN	BREAKFAST	LUNCH	DINNER	BEDTIME
before				
after				
meal / other				

NOTES: ....

....

....

....

....

WEEK OF: ....

MON	BREAKFAST	LUNCH	DINNER	BEDTIME
before				
after				
meal / other				

TUE	BREAKFAST	LUNCH	DINNER	BEDTIME
before				
after				
meal / other				

WED	BREAKFAST	LUNCH	DINNER	BEDTIME
before				
after				
meal / other				

THU	BREAKFAST	LUNCH	DINNER	BEDTIME
before				
after				
meal / other				

FRI

	BREAKFAST	LUNCH	DINNER	BEDTIME
before				
after				
meal / other				

SAT

	BREAKFAST	LUNCH	DINNER	BEDTIME
before				
after				
meal / other				

SUN

	BREAKFAST	LUNCH	DINNER	BEDTIME
before				
after				
meal / other				

NOTES:

WEEK OF: ....

MON	BREAKFAST	LUNCH	DINNER	BEDTIME
before				
after				
meal / other				

TUE	BREAKFAST	LUNCH	DINNER	BEDTIME
before				
after				
meal / other				

WED	BREAKFAST	LUNCH	DINNER	BEDTIME
before				
after				
meal / other				

THU	BREAKFAST	LUNCH	DINNER	BEDTIME
before				
after				
meal / other				

FRI

	BREAKFAST	LUNCH	DINNER	BEDTIME
before				
after				
meal / other				

SAT

	BREAKFAST	LUNCH	DINNER	BEDTIME
before				
after				
meal / other				

SUN

	BREAKFAST	LUNCH	DINNER	BEDTIME
before				
after				
meal / other				

NOTES:

WEEK OF: ....

MON	BREAKFAST	LUNCH	DINNER	BEDTIME
before				
after				
meal / other				

TUE	BREAKFAST	LUNCH	DINNER	BEDTIME
before				
after				
meal / other				

WED	BREAKFAST	LUNCH	DINNER	BEDTIME
before				
after				
meal / other				

THU	BREAKFAST	LUNCH	DINNER	BEDTIME
before				
after				
meal / other				

FRI	BREAKFAST	LUNCH	DINNER	BEDTIME
before				
after				
meal / other				

SAT	BREAKFAST	LUNCH	DINNER	BEDTIME
before				
after				
meal / other				

SUN	BREAKFAST	LUNCH	DINNER	BEDTIME
before				
after				
meal / other				

OTES:

NOTES:

NOTES:

NOTES:

NOTES:

NOTES:

Made in the USA
Middletown, DE
26 October 2023